Essential Oils for Sore Throat

Essential Oil Recipes for
Sore Throat
for Diffusers, Roller Bottles,
Inhalers & more.

Rica V. Gadi

This book is dedicated to all the strong people who are taking responsibility of your own well being and doing something to be better.

All my heartfelt gratitude to the following people: my mom Ruby Jane, you have made me everything I am today; my dad Nestor-- my eternal, my angel, and the source of my perseverance; Mommyling, my spiritual guide ; Ria & Joe, the true witnesses of my transformation and my foundation pillars; Ellie Jane, the sparkle of our eyes;

Juan, thanks for always encouraging me to push harder - you are my ONE; Rocco & Radha, my reason for everything.

The Love of my family and friends is the fountain of inspiration that never runs dry. Thank you for constantly inspiring me, motivating me, and loving me unconditionally.

This book will never be complete without the help of my trusted and talented friends the #NOWsuperstars and my #oilbularya friends

Blending Essential Oils to use for a very specific reason has become very popular in the recent years. There are several reasons why this is so. Blending EOs is basically about inhaling - as it has been proven that aromas have the ability to trigger feelings, emotions and personal memories.

With this in mind, it is obvious that everyone is unique when it comes to what triggers your senses. It all boils down to personal preference for the aroma to trigger what you want to unleash. Everyone is different and we all connect to the aroma differently, so what might work for one might not work for another person.

Of course, we also want the blend we personalize to be therapeutic. This is the best reason why to blend essential oils. We want the blend we create to help us with a very specific emotion or physical condition. As much as smelling good is important in a blend, it is more important that we blend oils that is not only pleasing to the smell but also produces the therapeutic effect we are after.

Then you have to think about contraindications. Making sure the blend you create is safe to use.

I suggest that before blending find out if the oils you are using is safe for a condition you may have example, if you are pregnant, or have specific allergies. Consult your physician prior to moving forward.

The recipes I have in this book is a compilation of what has proven to work and favored by hundreds of EO enthusiasts. It takes out the guesswork to get you started.

Again, we urge you to read the recipes and make sure that this is safe for you to try.

The book is very specific to a physical and emotional condition. There are several recipes here because you might want to rotate and you may like one and not the other. There is also a variety of application. Some of us prefer to diffuse, some to make roller bottles, and others to create sprays.

I hope you enjoy this compilation, feel free to use the notes section and jot down your fave blends. There is a wonderful world of EO blending - this is just the beginning.

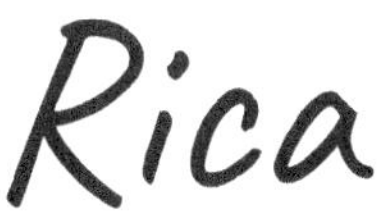

When a cold is about to come, sore throats are usually the first indicator of its arrival. They are mostly caused by bacteria or a virus. When they are viral, they are often with other symptoms of cold such as cough, runny nose, watery or reddish eyes and a whole lot of sneezing. Some other causes of sore throat may also include irritants in the air, pollution, allergies, dry air or smoking.

Sore throats are usually a symptom to an illness. There is nothing to worry about sore throats as it is normally caused a cold or your seasonal flu germs. In very rare occasions, a sore throat is also the first sign of being infected with the very scary ebola virus.

You should also seek medical attention when a sore throat is accompanied by other symptoms like rashes, tummy aches and a fever as it could also be a sign of strep.

Essential oils can help for sore throat by boosting your immune system, preventing the spreading of it to people around you and not to mention calming the discomfort that come along with it. EOs can help relieve inflammation and pain brought on by the infection and get you off to start the healing process.

Table of Contents

Best Essential Oils for Sore Throat

Having a cold or cough is definitely no fun at all. Not only because you will endure the excruciating pain on your throat but you will wake yourself up every time you sleep due to consistent coughing and the worst case scenario is that you will unknowingly spread the virus and might affect other people around you.

Sore throat or medically termed as pharyngitis is a common bacterial or viral infection that gets out from nowhere and affects all people easily since it's very contagious. It usually starts with flu or a cold and slowly by slowly you will have this itchy feeling on your throat and then involuntary movements of your throat such as swallowing will be painful, all of these instances   are usually caused by allergies, smoking and acid reflux.

When a sore throat occurs, you will definitely look for tablets or pain relievers to ease the pain on your throat and some rushes directly to the doctor for antibiotics. But you don't need to worry and wait for your sore throat to go away and become hopeless because aside from the normally recommended proper nutrition, drinking a tantamount of liquids and rest, one of the best remedies that have been identified is the use of essential oils for sore throat. By using these oils for your swollen throat, it kills bacteria and viruses to prevent the spread of the disease and boosts your immune system. Below is the list of essential oils that are deemed effective enough to cure sore throat.

Peppermint Essential Oil

Peppermint Essential Oil contains antimicrobial and decongestant properties that can easily alleviate the pain most especially in soothing throats. Its main component is menthol, an active ingredient that provides a cooling effect and a calming sensation to the body. To make use of peppermint oil's fullest capacity, you can mix it with carrier oil and rub it on the skin specifically on your throat and chest. You can also add the peppermint oil on a vaporizer for aromatherapy or to a soothing tea. In that way, you can definitely calm yourself from the itchy feeling and any movement of your muscles on the throat will go smoothly.

Eucalyptus Essential Oil

Though eucalyptus appears to be in many pharmacies and over the counters in a form of syrup, tablets or a soothing wax still Eucalyptus as an essential oil for your swollen throat is a great way to relieve the pain since it's known for its capability to stimulate the pain and provide protection against viral or bacterial infections that leads to sore throat. Eucalyptus contains cineole, an organic compound that reduces inflammation and pain. To make use of eucalyptus essential oil, you can add 1-2 drops to a humidifier or bath water or you can add 1-2 drops of eucalyptus oil to a cup of water and then gargle then absolutely it can easily inhibit the growth of viruses on your throat and fight off infection faster.

Thyme Essential Oil

Thyme oil is known to be one of the strongest antioxidants and antimicrobials. During the ancient times, it has been used as a medicinal herb since it greatly supports the immune and respiratory system. It has a capacity to sooth muscle spasms that leads to sore throat. To get the fullest capacity of thyme as an essential oil for sore throat, you can dilute it with a carrier oil, can be taken orally, or you can apply it to the affected area on your neck or chest.

Lemon Essential Oil

Lemon is widely used in a lot of different ailments and diseases since it contains antibacterial properties. Using the skin of lemon, the oil is extracted to create lemon essential oil. It can easily cleanse toxins on any part of the body and is commonly used to rejuvenate the skin. It is also excellent in curing sore throat since it contains Vitamin C and also can easily keep the throat moist since it increases the production of a certain amount of saliva. To make use of it's full capacity, you can pour two to three drops of lemon essential oil on a diffuser since the lemon provides a soothing smell on a diffuser which is good for aromatherapy, can be used also as a gargle ingredient for easy use or you can add it on your tea.

Ginger Essential Oil

Ginger is a pungent spicy herb that has been usually used for healing and cooking purposes. But what's great about ginger is that it doesn't limit its own capacity since it has been scientifically proven that it's very effective for sore throat. Ginger as an essential oil for sore throat has been tagged as one of the most recommended oils to be used since it provides relief to the swollen throat; it also boosts immunity as it fights an infection that causes sore throats. Ginger essential oil is best used to incorporate it with your tea because it is the best home remedy for sore throat, two to three times of drinking tea would be enough to get away with the inflammation on your throat.

Essential Oils are truly popular nowadays as an alternative remedy for sore throat as it has proven that these oils contain antibacterial and anti-inflammatory properties. As soon as you feel like the symptoms of sore throat such as scratchiness and the difficulty of swallowing do not hesitate to use any preventive measures to alleviate the symptoms by using essential oils to easily prevent or shorten the duration by reducing the pain and inflammation. Definitely, you can never go wrong by using these highly recommended essential oils.

It is also worth mentioning that the following oils are worth checking out for Sore Throat : **Tea Tree, Oregano, Cinnamon, Cedarwood, Ginger, Lavender and Rosemary**

The Blending Process

These EOs are categorized by aromas, and EOs from the same group usually blend fantastically together.

- Floral – Lavender, Geranium, Jasmine
- Woodsy – Pine, Cedarwood
- Earthy – Vetiver, Patchouli
- Herbaceous – Marjoram, Rosemary, Basil
- Minty – Peppermint, Spearmint, Wintergreen
- Medicinal – Eucalyptus, Frankincense, Melaleuca
- Spicy – Pepper, Clove, Cinnamon
- Oriental – Ginger, Patchouli
- Citrus – Wild Orange, Lemon, Lime

Select oils that will give you with the health benefits you are looking to remedy. For increased energy choose: Grapefruit, Lemon, Orange, or Citrus. For Calming and Relaxation choose: Lavender, Cedarwood, or Chamomile. You are encouraged to experiment and play with your oils to see which blends work for you.

TIPS:

- Combine Floral EOs with Woodsy, Spicy and Citrus aromas
- Minty EOs with Woodsy, Earthy, Herbaceous and Citrus aromas
- Earthy EOs with Woodsy and Minty aromas
- Citrus EOs with Floral, Woodsy, Minty, Spicy and Oriental aromas

Diffuse

Diffusing Essential Oils is the safest method to enjoy Essential Oils without the risk of an allergic reaction.

Diffusing Essential Oils
Some Tidbits You Need To Know

Our sense of smell is one of our most powerful senses, and as you have noticed in your own experience that some scents affect your more positively in your minds than others. The body contains over 1,000 receptors for smell—way more receptors than for any of our other senses.

Diffusion Essential Oils means the process vaporizes oils into air by releasing tiny amounts into the air. Inhalation is totally safe and is super low risk. Chances of any EO rising to dangerous levels while diffusion is slim to none.

Diffusing Essential Oils around newborns, babies, young children, pregnant or nursing women, and pets should be done with caution. Read up on safety.

It is advisable that Diffusing Essential Oils for only about 15-30 minutes at a time to be most effective. NEVER leave your diffuser on overnight. Make sure your diffuser is filled with the right amount of water and you understand the operating directions.

While diffusing essential oils, be sure that your space has great ventilation. Crack a window open if the scent become to strong.

Never add Carrier Oils to your diffuser. This may cause your diffuser to malfunction. Clean your diffuser at least 3 times a week with warm water and natural soap to ensure the diffuser is well maintained and bacteria and mold does not accumulate.

Diffusing Essential Oils
Basic Guidelines

Just a few things you need to know and prepare before getting started Diffusing Essential Oils.

Things you need:
Ultrasonic Oil Diffuser
Essential Oils
Water

Just follow the number of drops in the recipe, drop on to an oil diffuser and fill the rest with water.

All diffusers are different and will have its own water minimum and maximum level. Read the diffuser instruction before use.

Ideally, it is best to diffuse for 15-30 minutes and turn off the diffuser. The effect should be good for at least 2-3 hours. Turn your diffuser back on after 3 hours to reinforce oil diffusing effects.

It is not advisable to use EO in humidifiers.

These are not made to release EOS

Diffuser Recipes

Here's a thought for you:

You may be wondering how aroma can simply eliminate symptoms. There's a simple answer to this : Aroma is simply a by-product of diffusing. It's the added benefit but in reality the real benefit comes from the air we breathe and how the body easily absorbs the essential oils released in the air. It works 2 ways, not only does it improve the air quality you breath by disinfecting and eliminating pollutants it also allows your glands to absorb the healing elements of the EOs released in the air molecules,

So for here are a few recipes that can help you manage symptoms and actual issues regarding the matter :

3 Drops Lemon
3 Drops Scotch Pine
3 Drops Lavender
1 Drop Peppermint

----

3 Drops Juniper Berry
4 Drops Rosemary
4 Drops Frankincense

----

4 Drops Cypress
6 Drops Grapefruit

----

5 Drops Cedarwood
4 Drops Lavender
1 Drop Chamomile
1 Drop Eucalyptus (optional)

5-7 Drops Pine or Cedarwood
5-7 Drops Lavender
4 Drops Eucalyptus
1 Drop Lemon

3-5 Drops Rosemary
2 Drops Thyme
1 Drop Peppermint

----

3 Drops Peppermint
3 Drops Lemon
3 Drops Eucalyptus

----

2 Drops Oregano
2 Drops Tea Tree
2 Drops Peppermint
2 Drops Lavender
2 Drops Lemon

3 Drops Tea Tree
2 Drops Lavender
2 Drops Peppermint

----

4 Drops Lavender
4 Drops Peppermint
2 Drops Frankincense
2 Drops Basil

----

3 Drops Rosemary
2 Drops Eucalyptus
2 Drops Peppermint
1 Drops Cypress
1 Drops Lemon
----

2 Drops Lemon
1 Drops Lime
2 Drops Peppermint
1 Drops Rosemary
2 Drops Eucalyptus
1 Drop Clove
----

3 Drops RC
3 Drops Lemon
3 Drops Purification
----

2 Drops Eucalyptus
1 Drops Peppermint

3 Drops Frankincense

----

4 Drops Thieves
3 Drops Eucalyptus Radiata
3 Drops Lavender

----

1 Drop Lemon
1 Drop Eucalyptus
2 Drops Peppermint
1 Drop Rosemary

----

1 Drop Rosemary
2 Drops Eucalyptus
2 Drops Lime
1 Drop Peppermint
1 Drops Frankincense

----

2 Drops Frankincense
2 Drops Orange
1 Drop Eucalyptus

2 Drops Oregano
2 Drops Rosemary
2 Drops Peppermint
2 Drops Eucalyptus

----

3 Drops Eucalyptus
2 Drops Lavender
2 Drop Peppermint

----

3 Drops Eucalyptus
3 Drops Tea Tree

----

4 Drops Eucalyptus
2 Drops Myrrh
4 Drops Cedarwood

----

4 Drops Eucalyptus
2 Drops Ginger
4 Drops Rosemary

----

4 Drops Tea Tree
4 Drops Eucalyptus

Roll

Essential Oil Roller Bottles is the easiest method to enjoy Essential Oils Anywhere and Whenever.

Blending Essential Oils in a Roller Bottle
Some Tidbits You Need To Know

Essential Oils are usually super concentrated and too hard to measure how much to actually put straight from the bottle.

Roller bottles are a way that you are able to create blends ready to use with the right dilution. It allows your EO to last longer.

It also makes it easier to apply exactly where you want to target without getting it all over the place.

It is handy and easy to carry in your purse, ready to use at any time you want to.

I like to apply EOs at the bottom of the feet for many reasons. Our feet have bigger pores than any other skin in our bodies. this means that they are able to suck in the therapeutic compounds in our blend into the bloodstream faster that any other parts of the body. Imagine comparing a normal straw to an oversized straw and how much more you can suck in with the latter. This is how the soles of our feet is compared to the rest of the skin in our bodies.

The skin on our feet is also less sensitive and is designed to withstand some abuse. The risk of having an irritation from EOS is less likely to happen when applied on the feet.

The feet don't have the glands that act as a barrier. Sebaceous glands are glands in our skin that produces an oily substance called Sebum, for the purpose of lubricating and waterproofing the skin. Since this is oil and if you put oil on top of oil, it can act as a barrier or it may slow down penetration.

The feet and palms of our hands are the only skin that don't have these, so it is ideal to apply Essential Oils to the feet for maximum penetration.

Now, it would be hard to apply oils directly and very mess, right? Roller bottles make it super easy and convenient to roll the EOs at the bottom of our feet.

Carrier Oils Info

Carrier oils are vegetable-based oils with their own healing properties that dilute essential oils used to help carry the EOs into the skin.

Essential oils are highly concentrated and could evaporate very quickly. The carrier oil is mixed with the essential oil so it could penetrate the skin before it actually evaporates. Although EOs are oils, it is actually not that oily. When mixed with a carrier oil, it allows you to have more of the essential oil into your skin without wasting EOS to evaporate, making the healing properties of the EO strong and more effective.

There are also Essential oils that are too strong to apply directly to the skin and may cause damage, so it is important to dilute them with a carrier oil.

Never add Carrier Oils to your diffuser. This may cause your diffuser to malfunction. Clean your diffuser at least 3 times a week with warm water and natural soap to ensure the diffuser is well maintained and bacteria and mold does not accumulate.

Carrier Oils

There are a lot of different carrier oils that you can use with EOs to dilute them in a roller bottle.

To name a few :

Almond Oil - moisturizing and stays liquid at room temperature. Do not use if you are allergic to nuts.

Apricot Kernel Oil - moisturizing and suitable for sensitive skin or kids. It is super gentle on the skin.

Avocado Oil - moisturizing and suitable for sensitive and damaged skin. Perfect for skin problems.Can be mixed with other carrier oils

Castor Oil - with antibacterial, antiviral and antifungal properties, use topically to eliminate pain and relieve skin irritation.

Coconut Oil - its antibacterial, antiviral and antifungal properties it is the best and most versatile for skin care. The skin absorbs this very quickly. It solidifies in room temp and may still have a slight coconut oil aroma in it - but you can get a fractionated coconut oil to eliminate the 2 challenges above.

Grapeseed Oil - not just for cooking but also great for topical application on the skin.

Jojoba Oil - one of my faves for skin care blends. This oil is the closest to our natural oil our skin produces to it is absorbed easily without being oily. Also amazing for massage oil blends.

Olive Oil - this is the oil for herb type oils. mostly used for cooking but can also be applied to the skin but would need to be blended with a carrier oil that is mild and absorb well with the skin.

Rosehip Seed Oil - super good for deep moisturizing or skin irritations. This oil has a high content of antioxidants and helps remedy dry, scarred and wounded skin.

Recommended Roller Bottle Dilution Guide

RECOMMENDED ROLL-ON BOTTLE DILUTION AMOUNTS

5 ml (1/6 oz.) Roll-on Bottle = ~100 drops (1tsp.)
10 ml (1/3 oz.) Roll-on Bottle = ~200 drops (2 tsp.)
30 ml. (1 oz.) Roll-on Bottle = ~600 drops (6 tsp.)

Roll-on Size	5 ml	10 ml	30 ml	Add EO drops to roll-on, then fill with carrier oil.	Dilution Percentage
	1	2	6	1%	
	2	4	12	2%	
	3	6	18	3%	
Essential Oil Drops	5	10	30	5%	
	10	20	60	10%	
	20	40	120	20%	
	25	50	150	25%	
	50	100	300	50%	

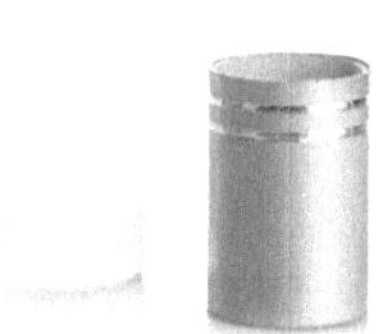

General Guidelines:
Birth to 12 months = .3-.5% dilution
1-5 years = 1.5-3% dilution
6-11 years = 1.5-5% dilution
12-17 years = 1.5-20% dilution
18 years and older = 1.5% dilution-Neat (no dilution)
Elderly or Sensitive Skin = 1-3% dilution
Daily Use = 2-5% dilution
Short Term Use = 10-25% dilution
Local Skin or Systemic Issues = 50% dilution-Neat

These are general guidelines suggestions--not absolute rules--based on traditional aromatheraphy practice.
(Kurt Schnaubelt PhD, Valerie Worwood, Robert Tisserand)

Dilution Basics:

How much you dilute your EO depends on different factors such as weight, sensitivity, health conditions, EOs that are blended in or how long that blend has been used for. There is never an absolute dilution rule, it is you who knows about your level and tolerance. I feel that it is best to start with a higher dilution percentage and increase EO drops over time.

To make sure your EO is safe, make sure that the oils you use are therapeutic grade and do your research on the source and extraction methods used to produce the oils.

Roller Bottle Blending Order

I normally just start with dropping the drops of oils into the **10mL roller bottle**, then adding the carrier oil up until the shoulder of the bottle. Capping the bottle off with the roller and the bottle cap. Instead of shaking the bottle, i like to roll the bottle between my palms first for a minute or 2 for blending, then finishing it off with a few shakes.

NOTE: All recipes in this book is for a 10mL Roller Bottle. If you have a bigger or smaller roller bottle, adjust the number of EO drops based on the size of your bottle.

Roller Bottle Recipes

4 drops Onguard
4 drops Oregano
4 drops Lemon

----

10 drops Respiratory Blend
6 drops Lime

----

5 drops Eucalyptus
3 drops Frankincense
2 drops Lemon

----

8 drops Breathe
5 drops Lime

----

6 drops Respiratory Blend
4 drops Eucalyptus
3 drops Frankincense

----

4 drops Lemon
4 drops Peppermint
2 drops Frankincense

----

6 drops RC
4 drops Lemon
4 drops Purification
2 drops Thyme

----

3 drops Lemon
3 drops Clove
3 drops Eucalyptus
3 drops Rosemary

----

4 drops Oregano
6 drops Lemon
5 drops On Guard
5 drops Melaleuca

----

4 drops Frankincense
4 drops Lemon
4 drops Melaleuca Tea Tree
4 drops Protective Blend

----

2 drops Oregano
2 drops Melaleuca
2 drops Lemon
2 drops Frankincense
2 drops Cinnamon

----

3 drops Orange
3 drops Lemon
3 drops Thieves
3 drops Frankincense

----

4 drops Thieves

4 drops Purification
4 drops Oregano

----

8 drops Respiratory Blend
5 drops Eucalyptus
4 drops Frankincense

----

6 drop Cardamom
6 drop Frankincense

----

2 drops Oregano
2 drops Tea Tree
2 drops Lemon
2 drops Frankincense
2 drops Cinnamon

----

4 drops Peppermint
2 drops Eucalyptus
2 drops Lemon
2 drops Rosemary

----

2 drops Lemon
6 drops Lavender
2 drops Peppermint

----

4 drops Peace & Calming
3 drops Lavender

3 drops Frankincense

Bonus Recipes

Pain Relief Massage Oil Favorite

60mL Jojoba Oil (cold pressed)
8 drops Lavender
8 drops Peppermint
15 drops Frankincense

Pain Relief Massage Oil Secret

14 drops Frankincense
10 drops Sweet Orange
8 drops Turmeric
30mL Sweet Almond Oil

Pain Relief Bath Soak Blend

10 drops Frankincense
5 drops Lavender
5 drops Bergamot
1 cup Full-Cream/ Full-Fat Milk

Pain Relief Bath Salt Blend

1 cup Epsom Salt
¼ cup Dead Sea Salt
¼ cup Baking Soda
8-10 drops Essential Oils
(use any ingredient above or single oils)

Inhale

Essential Oil Inhalers are the most convenient way to enjoy Essential Oils Anywhere and Whenever.

Essential Oil Inhalers give you quick and easy access to the vast therapeutic benefits of essential oils.

Blending Essential Oils in an Inhaler
Some Tidbits You Need To Know

EO Inhalers or aroma sticks are compact tubes, with a cotton wick inside and a protective cover, to lock the aroma within.

Your preferred blend of essential oils is absorbed by the cotton wick, and safely enclosed in a tube that that fits inside of the cover. The cover is easily removed for access to the tube to breathe in the aroma. Usually lasts about 3 months, depending on the oil blend used.

I absolutely love these because they encourage me to take a moment during super stressful moments, and just breathe.

It is in times of stress when our breathing patterns often change and taking deep breaths promote a feeling of calm and inner peace. Breath work combined with visualization plus a relaxing inhaler, can offer relief to symptoms of stress and help your body to come back to the state of homeostasis.

Aroma Sticks can be carried in your tiny purse, even compact enough to fit in your pocket. You can enjoy your favorite EOs anywhere and you can use them with discretion.

I love diffusing, and do all the time but not everyone in my space may enjoy the scents I enjoy or they may not benefit from the therapeutic benefits of the EOs I am diffusing - so the inhaler is one way to not only enjoy my choice of blends but to keep in personal not affecting everyone else around me.

Inhalers not only benefits me but also keep those around me safe in case the oils I want to blend may pose a risk to those around me who may have health issue not advised to be exposed to my choice EOs/

When making Aroma Sticks, You may use your chosen EOs at 100% Concentration.

Inhaler Basic Guidelines

Breathe in slow and deep to absorb the EO molecules directly into your olfactory system.

Inhalers are super easy to use. You just remove the cap and inhale from the inhaler tube, count 1 to 5 slowly as you inhale. The EO molecules get drawn into our bloodstream through our nasal cavity and gets delivered throughout our entire body.

Simple to use, easy to cary, portable and compact. You never have to be without your favorite blends, ever.

Inhaler Blending Basics

Inhalers are super easy and simple to make.

All you need is an inhaler set which consist of the following:

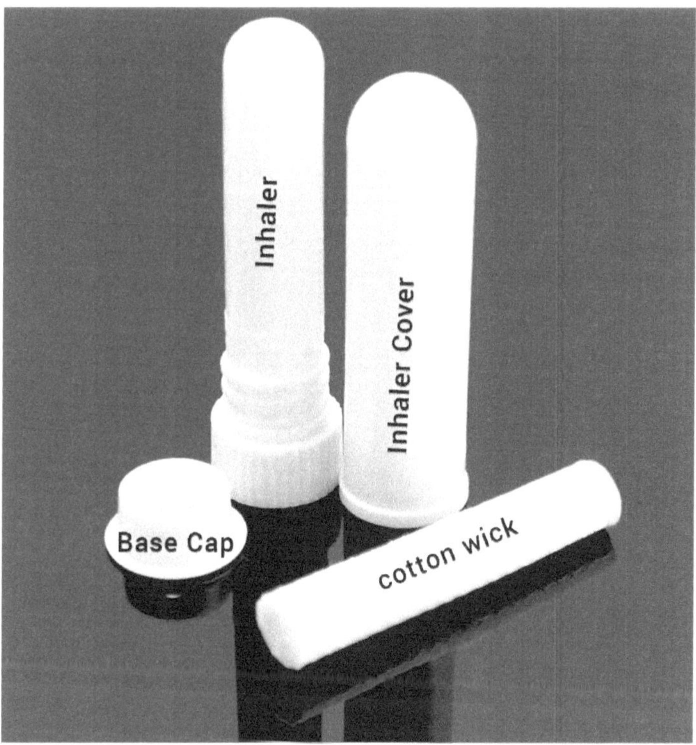

Inhaler, Inhaler Cover, Base Cap and Cotton Wick.

You will need your Essential Oils.

I like to use a pipette for precision and a small petri dish so I can see the oil.

Blending is super easy, just combine the drops and swirl it around in the petri dish and when you are satisfied you can go ahead and drop the cotton wick to absorb all the oil in the dish.

Once the wick is ready you can drop it in the inhaler and cap the bottom with the Base Cap. I usually like to secure the cover with the inhaler so I don't have to do it later.

I usually us 15-20 drops of EO total in a recipe and it can last up to 3 months. Some recipes will need more but on average it is in this range.

Inhaler Recipes

6 drops of Balance
4 drops of Eucalyptus
3 drops of Lemon
2 drops of Lime

----

5 drops of Frankincense
6 drops of Lavender
4 drops of Wild Orange

----

5 drops RC
2 drops Peppermint
2 drops Frankincense

----

3 drops of Lavender
3 drops of Lemon
3 drops of Melrose
3 drops of Eucalyptus
3 drops of RC
3 drops of Peppermint
3 drops of Copaiba

----

2 drop of Lemon
4 drops of Eucalyptus Radiata
6 drops of Rosemary
4 drops of Peppermint

----

4 drops of Peppermint
4 drops of Eucalyptus
2 drops of Lavender
2 drops of Lemon
2 drops of Rosemary

----

4 drops of Eucalyptus
4 drops of Siberian Fir
4 drops of Peppermint

----

9 drops Rosemary
3 drop Thyme
3 drop Peppermint

5-7 drops of Pine or Cedarwood
5-7 drops of Lavender
4 drops of Eucalyptus
1 drop of Lemon
----

8 drops of Rosemary
8 drops of Peppermint
6 drops of Eucalyptus
----

10 drops of Rosemary
4 drops of Thyme
2 drop of Peppermint
----

6 drops of Pine or Rosemary
6 drops of Peppermint
4 drops of Eucalyptus
----

9 drops of Rosemary
3 drop of Thyme
3 drop of Peppermint
----

3 drops of Oregano
3 drops of Tea Tree
3 drops of Lemon
3 drops of Frankincense
3 drops of Cinnamon Leaf
----

6 drops of Spruce
4 drops of Eucalyptus
3 drops of Lemon
2 drops of Lime
----

5 drops of Frankincense
6 drops of Lavender
4 drops of Wild Orange
----

6 drops of Eucalyptus
3 drops of Roman Chamomile
6 drops of Frankincense
----

4 drops of Cedarwood
6 drops of Roman Chamomile
10 drops of Frankincense
----

8 drops of Thieves
4 drops of Frankincense
4 drops of Lemon
----

5 drops of Lemon
5 drops of Lavender
5 drops of Peppermint
----

3 drops of Oregano
3 drops of Tea Tree
3 drops of Lemon
3 drops of Frankincense
3 drops of Cinnamon
----

9 drops of Hyssop
5 drops of Black Spruce
3 drops of Lavender
1 drop of Peppermint
----

3 drop of Black Spruce
6 drops of Lavender
6 drops of Scotch Pine
3 drop of Spearmint

Book Ordering

To order your copy / copies of

Essential Oils for Colds

please visit: **EOrecipes.net**

You can also check out other titles available.

Bulk Pricing and
Affiliate Programs Available